The Hemochromatosis Cookbook

A Comprehensive Guide To Managing Iron Absorption And Symptoms, Offering Easy-To-Follow Recipes For A Balanced Diet

Marjorie Champlin

Table of Contents

CHAPTER ONE

Introduction

Hemochromatosis is a genetic disorder characterized by excessive absorption and storage of iron in the body. Typically, the body regulates iron absorption based on its needs, but in individuals with hemochromatosis, this mechanism is disrupted, leading to an accumulation of iron in various organs and tissues.

There are two primary types of hemochromatosis:

Hereditary Hemochromatosis (HH): This is the most common form and is caused by genetic mutations that affect the regulation of iron absorption. The most prevalent mutations associated with HH are found in the HFE gene.

Secondary Hemochromatosis: This can occur due to other conditions like repeated blood transfusions, chronic liver disease, or excessive iron intake.

Symptoms may vary widely and can include fatigue, joint pain, abdominal pain, weakness, and bronze or grayish skin discoloration. However, some individuals might not exhibit noticeable symptoms for years, even though iron continues to accumulate in their organs.

If left untreated, hemochromatosis can lead to serious complications such as liver disease, heart problems, diabetes, and joint damage. Diagnosis often involves blood tests to measure iron levels and genetic testing to identify specific mutations associated with hereditary forms.

Treatment primarily focuses on reducing iron levels in the body by regularly removing blood through phlebotomy or iron chelation therapy. Additionally, dietary changes, such as avoiding iron supplements and limiting intake of iron-rich foods, may be recommended.

Early detection and management of hemochromatosis are crucial in preventing complications and maintaining overall health. Regular monitoring and adherence to treatment plans prescribed by healthcare professionals are essential for individuals with this condition.

Causes

Hemochromatosis has distinct causes and risk factors contributing to its development:

Genetic Factors:

Hereditary Hemochromatosis (HH): The most common form, caused by genetic mutations, particularly in the HFE gene. Mutations disrupt normal iron regulation, leading to excessive iron absorption and storage.

Other genes, like HJV, HAMP, and TFR, might also play a role in less common types of hereditary hemochromatosis.

Secondary Hemochromatosis:

Results from other conditions or factors:

Chronic Liver Disease: Conditions like hepatitis, alcoholic liver disease, or non-alcoholic fatty liver disease can disrupt iron regulation.

Repeated Blood Transfusions: Individuals reliant on frequent transfusions can accumulate excess iron due to the additional iron introduced via transfusions.

Excessive Iron Intake: This can occur from high-dose supplements or certain dietary habits.

Risk Factors

Genetics: Having a family history of hemochromatosis significantly increases the risk, especially if a close relative has been diagnosed.

Ethnic Background: Certain populations, particularly those of Northern European descent, have a higher prevalence of hereditary hemochromatosis.

Gender: Men are more likely to develop symptoms and complications due to higher iron levels compared to premenopausal women, who regularly lose iron through menstruation.

Diagnosis

Diagnosing hemochromatosis involves a combination of clinical assessments, blood tests, genetic testing, and sometimes imaging studies. Screening for this condition is especially important for individuals with risk factors or a family history of hemochromatosis.

Physical Examination: The doctor may look for signs like skin discoloration, joint pain, or an enlarged liver or spleen.

Blood Tests:

Serum Iron Levels: Measures the amount of iron in the blood.

Transferrin Saturation: Determines the percentage of transferrin (a protein that transports iron) that is saturated with iron.

Serum Ferritin: Measures the body's iron stores.

Genetic Testing: Identifies specific mutations associated with hereditary hemochromatosis, especially if there's a family history or clinical suspicion.

Screening

Family History Assessment: Individuals with a family history of hemochromatosis are encouraged to undergo screening.

Risk Assessment: Doctors might recommend screening for individuals with symptoms suggestive of hemochromatosis or those at higher risk due to factors like ethnicity or known genetic predisposition.

Routine Check-ups: Regular check-ups that include blood tests for iron levels can help detect elevated iron levels before symptoms manifest.

CHAPTER TWO

Identifying Hemochromatosis

Identifying hemochromatosis involves recognizing its signs, conducting specific tests, and considering risk factors.

Signs and Symptoms:

Fatigue: Persistent tiredness and weakness.

Joint Pain: Especially in the hands and wrists.

Abdominal Pain: Discomfort in the upper right part of the abdomen.

Skin Discoloration: Bronze or grayish skin, particularly in sun-exposed areas.

Other Symptoms: Loss of libido, impotence (in males), and irregular menstruation (in females).

Screening Methods and Tests

Screening methods and tests for hemochromatosis aims to detect elevated iron levels or genetic mutations, especially in individuals with risk factors or a family history of the condition.

Laboratory Tests:

Serum Iron Levels: Measures the amount of iron circulating in the blood.

Elevated levels might indicate excessive iron absorption.

Transferrin Saturation: Calculates the percentage of transferrin (iron-carrying protein) that is saturated with iron. Elevated levels indicate increased iron absorption.

Serum Ferritin: Assesses the body's iron stores. Elevated levels suggest excess iron accumulation.

Genetic Testing:

Identifies specific mutations associated with hereditary hemochromatosis, especially in individuals with a family history or clinical suspicion. Testing for mutations in the HFE gene is common.

Imaging Studies:

MRI or CT Scan: These can evaluate iron levels in the liver or detect complications like cirrhosis or liver damage caused by iron overload.

Phlebotomy as a Treatment

Phlebotomy, commonly known as bloodletting, is a primary treatment for hemochromatosis. This therapeutic approach involves the controlled removal of blood from the body to reduce excessive iron levels.

Procedure:

Frequency: Initially, frequent sessions might be scheduled, often weekly or biweekly, until iron levels normalize.

Volume: The volume of blood removed during each session varies but typically ranges from to milliliters (about half a pint to a pint).

Monitoring: Blood tests are conducted regularly to track iron levels and determine the frequency of phlebotomy sessions required to maintain optimal iron levels.

Mechanism:

By removing blood, the body compensates by utilizing stored iron to generate new red blood cells. This leads to a gradual reduction in overall iron stores, effectively lowering excess iron levels in the body.

Benefits:

Phlebotomy is highly effective in rapidly reducing iron levels, thereby preventing or minimizing complications associated with iron overload.

It's relatively safe when performed by trained professionals, and the body quickly replenishes the lost blood.

Considerations:

The frequency and duration of phlebotomy sessions depend on individual iron levels and response to treatment.

Some individuals might experience temporary side effects like dizziness or fatigue after sessions, which typically resolve quickly.

Dietary and Lifestyle Changes

Dietary and lifestyle modifications play a supportive role in managing hemochromatosis and maintaining optimal iron levels. Here are some key considerations:

Iron-Rich Foods:

Limitation: Reducing consumption of iron-rich foods, such as red meat, liver, and iron-fortified foods, can help regulate iron intake.

Vitamin C and Iron Absorption:

Caution: Foods high in vitamin C can enhance iron absorption. Limiting the intake of vitamin C-rich foods or supplements when consuming meals that are high in iron can help moderate absorption.

Alcohol and Iron Absorption:

Moderation: Excessive alcohol consumption can exacerbate liver damage in individuals with hemochromatosis. Moderation or abstinence is advisable.

Calcium and Phytates:

Incorporation: Calcium-rich foods or those containing phytates (found in whole grains and legumes) might modestly inhibit iron absorption. Including these foods might help moderate iron uptake.

Iron Supplements:

Avoidance: Unless specifically prescribed by a healthcare professional, avoid iron supplements as they can exacerbate iron overload.

Hydration:

Adequate Fluid Intake: Maintaining proper hydration supports overall health and blood circulation but doesn't directly impact iron levels.

Regular Exercise:

Healthy Lifestyle: Regular physical activity supports overall health but doesn't directly affect iron levels in hemochromatosis.

CHAPTER THREE

Medications and Therapies

In managing hemochromatosis, medications and therapies are used to complement primary treatments like phlebotomy and dietary modifications, particularly in cases where those methods might not be sufficient or tolerated well:

Iron Chelation Therapy:

Purpose: Iron chelators are medications that bind to excess iron in the body, facilitating its removal through urine or stool.

Usage: Used when phlebotomy isn't viable or effective. Examples include deferasirox, deferiprone, and deferoxamine.

Hepatoprotective Medications:

Purpose: For individuals with hemochromatosis-related liver damage or cirrhosis, medications may be prescribed to support liver health and function.

Usage: Medications aimed at managing liver complications might include antioxidants or specific drugs targeting liver conditions.

Symptom Management:

Pain Relief: Over-the-counter or prescribed medications to manage joint pain or discomfort associated with hemochromatosis symptoms.

Genetic Counseling:

Guidance: While not a direct therapy, genetic counseling provides information about inheritance patterns, family planning, and the potential risk of passing on the condition to offspring.

Monitoring and Supportive Therapies:

Regular Monitoring: Continual monitoring of iron levels and overall health status is crucial for timely adjustments to treatment plans.

Supportive Therapies: Counseling, physical therapy, and support groups can help individuals cope with the emotional and physical aspects of living with hemochromatosis.

Research and Emerging Therapies:

Ongoing Studies: Scientists continue to explore new therapies and treatment options for hemochromatosis, including targeted gene therapies and novel approaches to manage iron overload.

Managing Complications

Managing complications associated with hemochromatosis involves addressing conditions that can arise due to excessive iron accumulation in various organs. Key complications and their management include:

Liver Disease:

Treatment: Managing liver complications might involve lifestyle changes, medications to support liver health, and, in severe cases, interventions to address cirrhosis or liver failure.

Heart Problems:

Monitoring and Treatment: Regular cardiac evaluations to monitor heart function and manage complications like cardiomyopathy or arrhythmias.

Diabetes:

Management: Controlling blood sugar levels through medication, diet, and lifestyle changes is crucial in individuals who develop diabetes due to hemochromatosis.

Joint Pain and Arthritis:

Pain Management: Pain relief medications, physical therapy, and lifestyle modifications to reduce joint discomfort.

Skin Changes:

Monitoring and Protection: Regular skin checks to monitor changes and protect the skin from sun exposure, which might exacerbate discoloration.

Endocrine Disorders:

Hormone Replacement: Addressing hormonal imbalances that might arise due to complications affecting the endocrine system.

Regular Monitoring and Follow-ups:

Continual Assessment: Ongoing monitoring of iron levels, organ function, and overall health to detect and manage complications promptly.

Managing complications involves a multidisciplinary approach, often involving hepatologists, cardiologists, endocrinologists, rheumatologists, and other specialists. Individualized treatment plans tailored to address specific complications help improve quality of life and minimize the impact of hemochromatosis-related conditions on overall health. Regular communication and coordination among healthcare providers are crucial for comprehensive care and management of complications.

Addressing Organ Damage

Addressing organ damage caused by hemochromatosis requires a targeted approach based on the affected organs:

Liver Damage:

Lifestyle Changes: Limiting alcohol consumption and maintaining a healthy diet.

Medications: Prescribed to manage liver complications or support liver function.

Regular Monitoring: Periodic liver function tests and imaging studies to assess liver health.

Heart Complications:

Cardiac Evaluation: Regular assessments to monitor heart function and manage complications like cardiomyopathy or arrhythmias.

Heart-Healthy Lifestyle: Adopting heart-healthy habits, such as maintaining a balanced diet and regular exercise, to support cardiac health.

Diabetes Management:

Blood Sugar Control: Careful management of blood sugar levels through medication, diet, and exercise to mitigate the impact of diabetes related to hemochromatosis.

Joint and Bone Health:

Pain Management: Medications, physical therapy, and lifestyle modifications to alleviate joint pain and discomfort.

Monitoring: Regular assessments to monitor joint health and bone density.

Endocrine System:

Hormone Replacement: Addressing hormonal imbalances through hormone replacement therapies, if necessary, due to complications affecting the endocrine system.

Skin Changes:

Sun Protection: Protecting the skin from sun exposure to prevent exacerbation of skin discoloration.

Dermatological Monitoring: Regular skin checks to monitor changes and address any concerns.

Addressing organ damage involves a comprehensive approach focusing on lifestyle modifications, targeted medications, regular monitoring, and interventions specific to the affected organs. Collaborative care involving various specialists ensures a holistic management strategy tailored to an individual's specific needs and organ involvement. Regular follow-ups and adjustments to treatment plans are essential to mitigate the impact of hemochromatosis on organ health.

CHAPTER FOUR

Handling Iron Overload-Related Conditions

Handling conditions arising from iron overload in hemochromatosis involves targeted approaches to mitigate the impact of excess iron on various bodily systems:

Phlebotomy:

Primary Treatment: Regular blood removal sessions to reduce iron levels and prevent complications associated with iron overload.

Iron Chelation Therapy:

Secondary Treatment: Using iron chelators to bind and remove excess iron from the body, especially in cases where phlebotomy might not be viable or sufficient.

Diet and Lifestyle Modifications:

Limiting Iron Intake: Avoiding iron supplements and moderating consumption of iron-rich foods to prevent further iron accumulation.

Balanced Diet: Emphasizing a balanced diet to support overall health while managing iron intake.

Monitoring and Early Intervention:

Regular Check-ups: Frequent monitoring of iron levels and organ function to detect changes early and intervene promptly.

Timely Adjustments: Adjusting treatment plans based on regular assessments to maintain optimal iron levels and prevent complications.

Managing Complications:

Organ-Specific Management: Tailored approaches to manage complications in organs affected by iron overload, such as liver, heart, joints, and endocrine system.

Symptomatic Relief: Addressing symptoms associated with iron overload-related conditions, such as joint pain or fatigue.

Handling iron overload-related conditions in hemochromatosis involves a multifaceted approach focusing on reducing iron levels, managing complications, adopting healthy lifestyle habits, and regular monitoring to ensure timely interventions. Collaboration among healthcare providers is crucial to develop comprehensive treatment strategies based on an individual's specific needs and health status.

Genetic Counseling and Family Screening

Genetic counseling and family screening play vital roles in managing hemochromatosis:

Genetic Counseling:

Education: Provides information about the genetic basis of hemochromatosis, inheritance patterns, and the risk of passing on the condition to offspring.

Risk Assessment: Helps individuals understand their personal risk based on family history and genetic testing.

Family Planning: Assists in making informed decisions about family planning options and reproductive choices.

Family Screening:

Identifying At-Risk Relatives: Encourages family members to undergo genetic testing or screening to determine their risk of hemochromatosis.

Early Detection: Facilitates early detection of the condition in at-risk family members, allowing for timely intervention and management.

Importance of Screening:

Early Intervention: Identifying individuals at risk allows for early intervention, reducing the likelihood of complications associated with undiagnosed hemochromatosis.

Preventive Measures: Allows for the implementation of preventive measures, such as lifestyle modifications or regular monitoring, in at-risk individuals.

Genetic counseling and family screening are essential components in managing hemochromatosis. They empower individuals and families with information about the condition, aid in risk assessment, and enable early detection and intervention, ultimately contributing to better outcomes and improved management of this genetic disorder.

Lifestyle Recommendations

Lifestyle recommendations for managing hemochromatosis focus on supporting overall health and moderating iron levels. Here are some key lifestyle guidelines:

Diet Modifications:

Limit Iron Intake: Reduce consumption of iron-rich foods like red meat, liver, and iron-fortified products.

Moderate Vitamin C: Vitamin C enhances iron absorption, so consider moderating intake when consuming meals high in iron.

Hydration and Alcohol:

Adequate Hydration: Maintain proper hydration, although it doesn't directly impact iron levels.

Limit Alcohol: Excessive alcohol can exacerbate liver damage. Moderation or abstinence is advisable.

Calcium and Phytates:

Include Moderately: Foods rich in calcium or phytates (found in whole grains and legumes) might modestly inhibit iron absorption.

Iron Supplements:

Avoid Unless Necessary: Refrain from taking iron supplements without specific medical guidance as they can worsen iron overload.

Regular Exercise:

Overall Health: Engage in regular physical activity for overall well-being, but it doesn't directly impact iron levels in hemochromatosis.

Regular Monitoring and Healthcare Visits:

Adherence to Follow-ups: Attend regular healthcare visits for monitoring iron levels and overall health status.

Sun Protection:

Skin Care: Protect skin from excessive sun exposure to minimize skin discoloration associated with hemochromatosis.

Adopting a balanced diet, moderation in alcohol consumption, regular physical activity, and adherence to healthcare follow-ups are key lifestyle recommendations. These adjustments support overall health and aid in managing iron levels in individuals affected by hemochromatosis. Always consult healthcare professionals for personalized guidance based on individual health needs.

CHAPTER FIVE

Exercise and Healthy Living

Exercise and healthy living are beneficial for individuals with hemochromatosis, supporting overall well-being despite not directly impacting iron levels. Here's how:

Regular Exercise:

Cardiovascular Health: Engage in regular aerobic exercise, like walking, cycling, or swimming, to support heart health and overall fitness.

Strength Training: Incorporate strength training exercises to build muscle strength and maintain bone health.

Balanced Lifestyle:

Healthy Diet: Follow a balanced diet, emphasizing fruits, vegetables, whole grains, and lean proteins.

Adequate Hydration: Ensure proper hydration for overall health.

Stress Management:

Stress Reduction: Practice stress-reducing techniques like meditation, yoga, or mindfulness to manage stress levels.

Avoidance of Risky Behaviors:

Moderate Alcohol: If consumed, do so in moderation to minimize its impact on liver health.

Sun Protection: Protect skin from excessive sun exposure to prevent skin damage.

Healthcare Follow-ups:

Regular Check-ups: Adhere to scheduled healthcare visits for monitoring iron levels and overall health status.

While exercise and healthy living don't directly affect iron levels in hemochromatosis, they contribute to overall well-being. Regular physical activity, a balanced diet, stress management, and avoiding risky behaviors support optimal health and improve quality of life for individuals managing this condition. Always consult healthcare professionals before starting any new exercise regimen or making significant lifestyle changes.

Conclusion

Living with hemochromatosis necessitates a multifaceted approach involving education, lifestyle modifications, healthcare collaboration, emotional support, and self-advocacy. Understanding the condition, managing iron levels through treatments like phlebotomy or chelation, and adopting a balanced lifestyle are crucial.

Additionally, seeking emotional support from loved ones or support groups, prioritizing mental health, and engaging in stress-relieving activities contribute to overall well-being. Each individual's journey with hemochromatosis is unique, but with the right strategies and support networks, managing the condition becomes more manageable. Through education, proactive healthcare participation, and emotional resilience, individuals affected by hemochromatosis can lead fulfilling lives while effectively managing their health.

THE END